contents

This guide is based on the view that the discipline of mental health nursing occurs within a primary health care framework and in partnership with consumers. Within this worldview, mental illness is seen as only a part of the person, with recovery from mental illness the aim. A *recovery* approach is the hallmark of contemporary models of mental health nursing care.

The guide has been designed as a quick reference for students and beginning practitioner mental health nurses. It is not intended to be a replacement for a more comprehensive mental health text or to override a mental health nurse's accountability or compliance with professional regulatory or organisational policies. Additional generic medication safety information has been included to support the mental health nurse in clinical practice. (ACMHN, <www.acmhn.org>)

Recovery and recovery-oriented practice[1]

The concept of *recovery* emerged from the consumer movement in the 1970s and 1980s and continues to be utilised and further developed by people with lived experience.

Recovery-oriented practice describes an approach to mental health care that encompasses principles of self-determination and individualised care. A recovery approach emphasises hope, social inclusion, goal-setting and self-management, and includes the following principles:

- self-direction and self-determination
- empowerment of consumers
- individualised and person-centred care
- holistic and integrated care
- non-linear journeys of personal growth and healing
- strengths-based approaches
- peer support.

■ RECOVERY 'STAR'[2]

The Star symbol was designed to reinforce the five common elements identified as necessary in supporting individual people with their recovery.

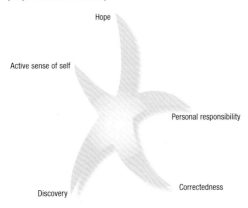

Hope

Active sense of self

Personal responsibility

Discovery

Correctedness

Mental state examination (MSE)

The MSE is an important part of the clinical assessment. It is a structured, systematised way of observing and then describing a consumer's current emotional state and physical appearance. Specific domains guide the MSE. These are appearance and behaviour, mood, affect, speech, thought form, thought content perception, insight/judgement and cognition.

■ KEY AREAS OF ASSESSMENT

DOMAINS	ISSUES TO EXPLORE
Appearance and behaviour	What does the consumer's grooming, posture, clothing, height and weight, psychomotor activity, mannerisms and gait look like?
Mood	What the consumer actually describes about how they are feeling—e.g. I feel depressed, I am really elated (subjective).
Affect	What you (the nurse) observe—e.g. the consumer appears perplexed, their affect is blunted (objective).
Speech	What is the consumer's speech like? Assess the rate, volume and flow—e.g. is it pressured speech, loud, quiet?
Thought form	Are the consumer's thoughts coherent—e.g. continuity of ideas, tangential, disturbance in language or meaning?
Thought content	What is the consumer actually thinking about—e.g. delusions, suicidal thoughts, obsessions, phobias?
Perception	Is the consumer admitting to or demonstrating signs of hallucinating or having illusions?

DOMAINS	ISSUES TO EXPLORE
Insight/ judgement	Does the consumer have an awareness and understanding of their illness? Can the person describe the early warning signs that they are becoming unwell? What illness does the consumer think they have? What triggers their illness? What does the consumer think is wrong? What brought them to seek help?
Cognition	Is the consumer oriented to time, place and person? What is their short-term and long-term memory like? Can they concentrate? For how long? Can they think in an abstract manner?
Risk	Is the consumer at risk of self-harm? Is anyone else at risk of harm from the consumer? Is there a risk of dependence or institutionalisation?

Self-harm risk assessment

■ ASSESSING FOR POTENTIAL RISK OF SUICIDE

- Is there a history of suicide attempts or self-mutilation?
- Is there a family history of suicide attempts or completion?
- Is there presence or a history of a mood disorder, or drug or alcohol misuse?
- Does the consumer have a mental illness (depression, schizophrenia, bipolar disorder)?

- Does the consumer have a history of chronic physical illness, chronic pain or recent surgery?
- Does the consumer have thoughts about harming self?
- To what extent does the consumer feel hopeless?

Example of how an MSE might be documented in nursing notes

Appearance and behaviour

Farid is a 31-year-old Lebanese/Australian man of average height and weight. At the time of the interview, he was well groomed and dressed neatly and casually in clean jeans and polo shirt. During the interview, Farid displayed no signs of tremor or abnormal movements. Farid was cooperative and pleasant, answering all questions without hesitation. Eye contact was maintained throughout the interview and posture was upright. He smiled appropriately during the interview. Farid's behaviour changed when he started talking about his brother. He became agitated and moved about in his seat. He also started to fiddle with his hands. He said that speaking about his brother, who had died from cancer, made him really sad. Farid said that it was the anniversary of his brother's death in one week.

Mood: When Farid was asked how he felt, he said that he was 'depressed'. He stated he 'wanted to die' and that he 'did not see what there was to look forward to'. He said, 'I would be better off dead.'

Affect: For the most part, Farid displayed a poor range of emotions during the interview. He did not look depressed. His affect changed when speaking of his brother. He became physically agitated, wringing his hands and was unable to sit still.

Speech: Farid articulated himself clearly. He answered questions spontaneously at a normal rate and rhythm. He spoke evenly throughout the conversation, except when he started to speak about his brother. At this time he spoke more loudly and more quickly.

Thought form: Farid did not exhibit any formal thought disorders. He was able to answer questions spontaneously and directly. He did not use any new or created words. Farid did experience thought block when exploring sensitivities in his past, particularly related to the death of his brother. No negative thought disorder was apparent.

Thought content: Farid was anxious about his physical health. He was obsessed with knowing his blood results and was constantly asking to see them. Thoughts that the tiredness was related to cancer were causing Farid to lack motivation and feel depressed. Other than appearing obsessed regarding blood results, Farid has no other positive symptoms, such as delusions, phobias or compulsions.

Perception: Perceptual disturbances were not noted during the MSE. Symptoms, such as illusions, misinterpretations, depersonalisation, passivity phenomena, were not elicited. There was also no indication of alterations to sensory perception. Farid denied any symptoms related to auditory, gustatory, olfactory, tactile or visual hallucinations.

Insight and judgement: When questioned about his condition, Farid accepted the fact that he is ill and that he requires treatment. He did not feel as though anything would work as he was 'too depressed' but was cooperative and was compliant with management.

Cognition: Farid was alert and orientated to person, time and place. He was able to answer questions and recall his past without difficulties.

Risk: Suicidal ideation was not detected, and his risk of self-harm was assessed as being low. Farid was asked if he wanted to harm himself and or others—he said no.

Mental illness: An overview[3]

The following lists give a quick overview of issues related to mental illness and mental health.

Statistics from the 2007 National Survey of Mental Health and Wellbeing[a]

- Almost half the total population (45.5%) experience a mental health disorder at some point in their lifetime.
- One in five, or 20% of the Australian population aged 16–85 years, experienced mental disorders in the previous 12 months [of their survey]. This is equivalent to 3.2 million Australians.
- One in 16 (6.2%) had affective (mood) disorders; one in seven (14.4%) had anxiety disorders; and one in 20 (5.1%) had substance abuse disorders.

- Based on these prevalence rates, it is estimated that nearly one million Australians have affective disorders; over 2.3 million had anxiety disorders and over 800 000 had substance use disorders in the previous 12 months.
- The prevalence of mental disorders declines with age: from 1 in 4 young people (16–24) to 1 in 20 (75–85 years).
- Only one third of people (34.9%) with a mental health disorder used health services for their mental health problem—and two thirds of people with a mental health disorder did not report using services for their mental health disorder.

Further statistics

- Depression and anxiety are the most prevalent mental disorders experienced by Australians. Depression alone is predicted to be one of the world's largest health problems by 2020.[b]
- Around one million Australian adults and 100 000 young people live with depression each year. On average, one in five people will experience depression in their lives; one in four females and one in six males.[c]
- Among young Australians aged 12–25 years, depression is the most common mental health problem. Around on-in-ten young Australians will experience an anxiety disorder in any given 12-month period.[d]
- At least one third of young people have had an episode of mental illness by the age of 25 years.[e]
- Mental disorders and suicide account for 14.2% of Australia's total health burden—which equates to 374 541 years of healthy life lost (DALYs).[f]

- Estimates suggest that up to 75% of people presenting with alcohol and drug problems also have additional mental health problems.[9]
- Reports indicate that up to 85% of homeless people have a mental illness.

■ DEFINITIONS

Affect	An expressed or observed emotional response—e.g. *restricted, flat or blunted.*
Compulsion	A strong, usually irresistible impulse to perform an act, especially one that is irrational or contrary to one's will—e.g. *repeated hand washing.*
Delusion	A fixed false belief that cannot be reasoned with or confronted with actual facts and that is not in keeping with the person's culture.
Hallucination	An alteration in sensory perception. Hallucinations can affect all five senses: —gustatory (taste) —visual (sight) —auditory (hearing) —tactile (touch) —olfactory (smell).

Illusion	A perception of stimuli that represents what is perceived in a way different from the way it is in reality—e.g. *shadow = robber, haze = water.*
Labile	Likely to change—e.g. *mood swings.*
Obsession	The domination of one's thoughts or feelings by a persistent idea—e.g. *feeling you are dirty.*
Psychosis	A general term used to describe a mental health problem in which a person has lost some contact with reality.

Signs of mental illness[4]

Having a mental illness often includes difficulty in thinking, socialising and functioning. These signs of mental illness are often arranged into six categories: thinking, feeling, socialising, functioning, problems at home and poor self-care.

These are symptoms of psychological disorders, and no symptom by itself is necessarily indicative of a mental illness. Two or three of these signs at one time may warrant further assessment. These signs of mental illness do not cover all the possible symptoms of mental illness. They are just the more common signs.

Thinking:
- difficulty concentrating, is easily distracted
- can't remember information

- processes information slowly, is confused
- has to work hard to solve problems
- can't think abstractly
- believes that there are messages on the TV, radio, computer or number plates that are specifically for them.

False or unusual perceptions:
- has perceptual distortions
- hallucinations: visual, tactile, gustatory, auditory, olfactory
- feels old situations are strangely new.

■ SYMPTOMS ASSOCIATED WITH DEPRESSION, MANIA AND ANXIETY

SYMPTOMS ASSOCIATED WITH DEPRESSION	SYMPTOMS ASSOCIATED WITH MANIA	SYMPTOMS ASSOCIATED WITH ANXIETY
Depressed mood	Impatient	Over-alert and on guard most of the time
Decreased appetite, weight loss	Overly confident and grandiose about abilities, talents, wealth, appearance	Feels anxious, afraid, and worried about everyday events
Difficulty sleeping, interrupted sleep, sleeping too much	Excessive energy; needs little sleep; no acknowledgement of fatigue	Avoids normal activities (taking the bus, grocery shopping)
Intrusive thoughts of death or suicide	Irritable much of the time	Uncomfortable around people

SYMPTOMS ASSOCIATED WITH DEPRESSION	SYMPTOMS ASSOCIATED WITH MANIA	SYMPTOMS ASSOCIATED WITH ANXIETY
Feeling worthless, hopeless and/or helpless	Speaks very fast, pressured speech, loud, difficult to interrupt	Compelled to do ritualistic or repeated behaviours
Feelings of guilt over minor things	Easily angered	Has upsetting, intrusive memories or nightmares of past events
Loss of interest and pleasure in most things	Excited, euphoric, overly confident, disruptive to others	
Difficulty with memory, concentration	Poor social judgement, engaging in reckless or self-destructive behaviour	
Difficulty with making decisions	Short attention span, easily distracted, loosened associations	
Wishing they were dead		

■ POSSIBLE SIGNS OF MENTAL HEALTH PROBLEMS

PROBLEMS WITH SOCIALISING	PROBLEMS WITH FUNCTIONING	PROBLEMS AT HOME	POOR SELF-CARE
Has few close friends	Gets fired or quits frequently	Can't attend to others' needs	Doesn't take care of appearance
Anxious and afraid around others	Is easily angered or irritated by normal stresses and expectations	Overwhelmed by chores or household responsibilities	Doesn't eat enough, or overeats
Verbally or physically aggressive	Can't get along with others at work, school or home	Can't keep up with housework	Doesn't take care of garden or home
Has tumultuous relationships, from overly critical to worshipful	Can't concentrate or work effectively	Instigates arguments and fights with family, passively or actively	Isn't attentive to cleanliness
Difficult to get along with	Can't meet expectations	Doesn't attend to finances, insurance bills, vehicle, etc.	
Can't read other people		Pays little or no attention to physical health	

Specific mental illnesses such as depression, bipolar, schizophrenia and anxiety disorders don't necessarily have symptoms that fall into one category. In other words, someone struggling with bipolar disorder could have signs of mental illness from each category (though there are some signs that are strictly bipolar, such as excessive energy and extreme mood swings).

Medications used in mental health

The medications listed below could be prescribed for a person living with mental illness.

Serum measures:

- µg/mL OR mcg/mL = microgram per millilitre
- ng/mL = nanogram per millilitre
- mEq/L = millilitre equivalent per litre
- mcmol = micromole.

GENERIC NAME	TRADE NAME	THERAPEUTIC SERUM LEVELS
Antipsychotics		
Aripiprazole	Abilify	
Chlorpromazine	Largactil	0.01–0.50 µg/mL
Clozapine	Clozaril	0.01–0.50 µg/mL
Fluphenazine	Modecate	
Haloperidol	Haldol	5–17 ng/mL
Iloperidone	Fanapt	

GENERIC NAME	TRADE NAME	THERAPUETIC SERUM LEVELS
Loxapine	Loxitane	0.01–0.03 µg/mL
Molindone	Moban	
Olanzapine	Zyprexa	0.009–0.023 µg/mL
Paliperidone	Invega	
Perphenazine	Trilafon	0.0004–0.0300 µg/mL
Pimozide (for Tourette's syndrome)	Orap	
Quetiapine	Seroquel	0.0004–0.0300 µg/mL
Risperidone	Risperdal	0.003–0.012 µg/mL
Thioridazine	Mellaril	0.1–2.6 µg/mL
Thiothixene	Navane	0.01–0.10 µg/mL
Trifluoperazine	Stelazine	0.5–2.0 µg/mL
Ziprasidone	Geodon	
Antidepressants (also for anxiety disorders)		
Alprazolam	Xanax, Niravam	
Amitriptyline (tricyclic) **RISK OF TOXICITY HIGH**	Elavil	120–150 ng/mL

GENERIC NAME	TRADE NAME	THERAPUETIC SERUM LEVELS
Bupropion	Wellbutrin	0.025–0.100 µg/mL
Citalopram (SSRI)	Celexa	0.081–0.16 µg/mL
Clomipramine (tricyclic) **RISK OF TOXICITY HIGH**	Anafranil	0.1–0.45 µg/mL
Desipramine (tricyclic) **RISK OF TOXICITY HIGH**	Norpramin	150–300 ng/ml
Doxepin (tricyclic) **RISK OF TOXICITY HIGH**	Sinequan	0.10–0.25 µg/mL
Duloxetine (SNRI)	Cymbalta	
Escitalopram (SSRI)	Lexapro	
Fluoxetine (SSRI)	Prozac	0.09–0.40 µg/mL
Fluvoxamine (SSRI)	Luvox	0.031–0.087 µg/mL
Imipramine (tricyclic) **RISK OF TOXICITY HIGH**	Tofranil	150–300 ng/mL
Isocarboxazid (MAOI)	Marplan	
Maprotiline (tricyclic) **RISK OF TOXICITY HIGH**	Ludiomil	0.05–0.718 µg/mL

GENERIC NAME	TRADE NAME	THERAPUETIC SERUM LEVELS
Mirtazapine	Remeron	0.039–0.18 µg/mL
Moxapine	Asendin	
Nortriptyline (tricyclic) **RISK OF TOXICITY HIGH**	Aventyl, Pamelor	0.05–0.375 µg/mL
Paroxetine (SSRI)	Paxil	0.031–0.062 µg/mL
Phenelzine (MAOI)	Nardil	0.001–0.002 µg/mL
Protriptyline (tricyclic)	Vivactil	0.07–0.38 µg/mL
Selegiline	Emsam	
Sertraline (SSRI)	Zoloft	0.055–0.25 µg/mL
Tranylcypromine (MAOI)	Parnate	
Trazodone	Desyrel	0.7–4.89 µg/mL
Trimipramine (tricyclic) **RISK OF TOXICITY HIGH**	Surmontil	0.01–0.30 µg/mL
Venlafaxine (SNRI)	Effexor	
Mood stabilising and anticonvulsants		
Carbamazepine	Tegretol	5–12 mg/L

GENERIC NAME	TRADE NAME	THERAPUETIC SERUM LEVELS
Divalproex sodium (valproic acid)	Depakote	
Gabapentin	Neurontin	2–10 µg/mL
Lamotrigine	Lamictal	1.5–3 mg/L
Lithium carbonate	Eskalith, Lithobid	0.8–1.2 mEq/L
Oxcarbazepine	Trileptal	
Phenytoin	Dilantin	10–20 µg/mL
Sodium valproate	Epilim	50–100 mg/L
Topiramate	Topamax	
Anxiolytics **(All the following are benzodiazepines, except Buspirone)**		
Alprazolam	Xanax	0.025–0.102 µg/mL
Buspirone	BuSpar	0.088–0.147 µg/mL
Chlordiazepoxide	Librium	0.67–3.1 µg/mL
Clonazepam	Klonopin	0.007–0.075 µg/mL
Clorazepate	Tranxene	0.1–1.6 µg/mL
Diazepam	Valium	0.31–6.00 µg/mL
Lorazepam	Ativan	0.01–0.24 µg/mL
Oxazepam	Serax	0.15–1.4 µg/mL

Neuroleptic malignant syndrome (NMS)

Neuroleptic malignant syndrome is a rare but potentially life-threatening reaction to the use of antipsychotic drugs or major tranquilisers (neuroleptics). See list of drugs associated with NMS.

Diagnostic criteria: Based on information from the DSM. 'The development of severe muscle rigidity and elevated temperature associated with the use of antipsychotic medication and two or more of the following:

* diaphoresis
* tremor
* dysphagia
* incontinence
* mutism
* tachycardia
* leucocytosis
* elevated or labile blood pressure
* changes in level of consciousness ranging from confusion to coma
* laboratory evidence of muscle injury (e.g. elevated creatine kinase (CK)).'[5]

■ MEDICATIONS ASSOCIATED WITH NMS[5]

GENERIC NAME	BRAND NAME
Chlorpromazine	Largactil
Haloperidol	Haldol
Loxapine	Loxitane

GENERIC NAME	BRAND NAME
Mesoridazine	serentil
Molindone	moban
Perphenazine	trilafon
Pimozide	orap
Thioridazine	mellaril
Thiothixene	navane
Trifluoperazine	stelazine
Atypical antipsychotics	
Aripiprazole	abilify
Clozapine	clozaril
Oolanzapine	zyprexa
Quetiapine	seroquel
Risperidone	risperdal
Ziprasidone	geodon
Dopamine antagonists	
Droperidol	Inapsine
Metoclopramide	reglan
Prochlorperazine	compazine
Promethazine	phenergan

■ EXTRA PYRAMIDAL SIDE EFFECTS (EPSE)

The extra pyramidal system is the nerves and muscles outside of the pyramidal tract and includes the nerve and muscle pathways involved in voluntary muscle movements. EPSE are a set of side effects that affect voluntary muscle movements.

ACUTE DYSTONIAS	PARKINSONISM	AKATHISIA	TARDIVE DYSKINESIA
Oculogyric crisis: 'look ups'—eyeballs spasm and lock into one position	Muscle rigidity	Feelings of restlessness	Involuntary blinking
Trismus: 'lockjaw'—jaw muscles clench, causing the jaw to lock	Tremor	Will feel as though they must move around	Eyebrow movement
Torticollis: tilted head—on one side of the neck the muscles contract abnormally	Slowed movement	Shift position frequently	Facial grimacing

Opisthotonus: entire body spasms—resulting in back arching and head and legs flexing back	Postural instability	Inability to stay still	Chorea—rapid, uncontrolled movements that look like the person is dancing
Macroglossia: tongue doesn't actually swell, but it protrudes and feels swollen			Involuntary spasms of the pelvis
TREATMENT[6] Dystonia responds well to anti-cholinergics (benztropine)	**TREATMENT[6]** Reduce the dose, replace with a different drug, add an anticholinergic	**TREATMENT[6]** Reduce the dose, replace with a different drug, add an anticholinergic	**TREATMENT[6]** No treatment for this side effect exists. PREVENTION!

Assessing specific mental health problems

■ PRE- AND POSTNATAL DEPRESSION[7]

The Edinburgh Postnatal Depression (PND) Scale is a set of questions designed to see if a new mother may have depression. The answers **will not provide a diagnosis**. The answers *will* tell you, however, whether the mother has symptoms that are common in women with PND.

To complete the set of questions, mothers should colour the circle next to the response which comes closest to how they have felt **in the past seven days**.

Scoring instructions: The total score is calculated by adding together the numbers circled for each of the ten items. The higher the score, the more likely it is that the person completing the questionnaire is distressed and may be depressed.

---

1. I have been able to laugh and see the funny side of things:
- ○ *0* As much as I always could
- ○ *1* Not quite as much now
- ○ *2* Definitely not so much now
- ○ *3* Not at all

2. I have looked forward with enjoyment to things:
- ○ *0* As much as I ever did
- ○ *1* Rather less than I used to
- ○ *2* Definitely less than I used to
- ○ *3* Hardly at all

3. I have blamed myself unnecessarily when things went wrong:
- ○ *3* Yes, most of the time
- ○ *2* Yes, some of the time
- ○ *1* Not very often
- ○ *0* No, never

4. I have been anxious or worried for no good reason:
- ○ *0* No, not at all
- ○ *1* Hardly ever
- ○ *2* Yes, sometimes
- ○ *3* Yes, very often

5. I have felt scared or panicky for no very good reason:
- ○ *3* Yes, quite a lot
- ○ *2* Yes, sometimes
- ○ *1* No, not much
- ○ *0* No, not at all

6. Things have been getting on top of me:
- ○ *3* Yes, most of the time I haven't been able to cope at all
- ○ *2* Yes, sometimes I haven't been coping as well as usual
- ○ *1* No, most of the time I have coped quite well
- ○ *0* No, I have been coping as well as ever

7. I have been so unhappy that I have had difficulty sleeping:
- ○ *3* Yes, most of the time
- ○ *2* Yes, sometimes
- ○ *1* Not very often
- ○ *0* No, not at all

8. I have felt sad or miserable:
- ○ *3* Yes, most of the time
- ○ *2* Yes, quite often
- ○ *1* Not very often
- ○ *0* No, not at all

9. I have been so unhappy that I have been crying:
- ○ *3* Yes, most of the time
- ○ *2* Yes, quite often
- ○ *1* Only occasionally
- ○ *0* No, never

10. The thought of harming myself has occurred to me:
- ○ *3* Yes, quite often
- ○ *2* Sometimes
- ○ *1* Hardly ever
- ○ *0* Never

PLEASE NOTE: This is a guide only. Clinical judgement forms an important part of any assessment and care. Scores apply to the **last seven days**. Use the guide in relation to the most recent Edinburgh Depression Scale (EDS).

SCORING SYSTEM:

Scores 0–9: May indicate the presence of some symptoms of distress that may be short-lived and are not likely to interfere with day-to-day ability to function at home or at work. However, if these symptoms have persisted more than a week or two, further enquiry is warranted as to the cause.

Scores 10–12: This range indicates the presence of symptoms of distress that may be discomforting. Repeat the EDS in one to two weeks' time; if the scores increase to 13 or above, assess further and consider referral to a mental health specialist.

Scores 13+: Scores of 13 or above require further evaluation and possible referral to a mental health specialist. Repeat the EDS at intervals to monitor progress.

*Item 10: Any woman who scores 1, 2 or 3 on item 10 requires further evaluation before leaving the unit/clinic to ensure her own safety and that of her baby.[8]

■ GERIATRIC DEPRESSION[9]

The Geriatric Depression Scale (short form) is shown below. Choose the best answer for how the consumer has felt over the past week.

1. Are you basically satisfied with your life?	YES / **NO**
2. Have you dropped many of your activities and interests?	**YES** / NO
3. Do you feel that your life is empty?	**YES** / NO
4. Do you often get bored?	**YES** / NO

5. Are you in good spirits most of the time?	YES / **NO**
6. Are you afraid that something bad is going to happen to you?	**YES** / NO
7. Do you feel happy most of the time?	YES / **NO**
8. Do you often feel helpless?	**YES** / NO
9. Do you prefer to stay at home, rather than going out and doing new things?	**YES** / NO
10. Do you feel you have more problems with memory than most?	**YES** / NO
11. Do you think it is wonderful to be alive now?	YES / **NO**
12. Do you feel pretty worthless the way you are now?	**YES** / NO
13. Do you feel full of energy?	YES / **NO**
14. Do you feel that your situation is hopeless?	**YES** / NO
15. Do you think that most people are better off than you are?	**YES** / NO

SCORING SYSTEM:

Score 1 for each **bolded** answer. A score >5 points is suggestive of depression and should warrant a further assessment. Scores >10 are almost always depression.

■ ASSESSING RISK OF SELF-HARM[10]

The following Sad Persons Scale is used to assess risk of self-harm.

S	**S**ex	Men kill themselves more often than women, but women make more attempts than men
A	**A**ge	High-risk groups <19 yrs; ≥45 yrs especially >65 yrs
D	**D**epression	Many people who attempt suicide have symptoms of depression
P	**P**revious attempts	65–70% of people who commit suicide have made previous attempts
E	**E**TOH	Alcohol is associated with up to 65% of successful suicides
R	**R**ational thinking loss	People who have lost touch with reality are more likely to commit suicide than the general population
S	**S**ocial support lacking	People with suicidal ideation often lack social supports (friends, family, meaningful work, spirituality or religion)
O	**O**rganised plan	Having a specific plan and the means to enact the plan are high-risk factors

| N | No spouse | People who are widowed, divorced, separated or single are at greatest risk—loneliness is a contributing factor |
| S | Sickness | Debilitating, chronic and severe illness |

SCORING SYSTEM:

Sex: 1 point if consumer is male, 0 if female

Age: 1 point if consumer is <19 yrs; ≥45 yrs especially >65 yrs

Depression: 1 point if consumer is depressed

Previous attempts: 1 point if yes

ETOH: 1 point if present

Rational thinking loss: 1 point if consumer is psychotic for any reason (schizophrenia, affective illness, organic brain syndrome)

Social support lacking: 1 point if these are lacking, especially with recent loss of a significant other

Organised plan: 1 point if plan made and method is lethal

No spouse: 1 point if divorced, widowed, separated or single (for males)

Sickness: 1 point, especially if chronic, debilitating, severe (e.g. non-localised cancer, epilepsy, multiple sclerosis, gastrointestinal disorders)

0–2: No real problems, keep watch

3–4: Send home, but check frequently

5–6: Consider admission, depending on level of assurance from consumer

7–10: Requires in-patient admission for own safety

Topics for psycho-education

Psycho-education is the sharing of information between mental health nurses and consumers and their families. Psycho-education empowers consumers to make informed decisions throughout their recovery journey. It is interactive—it is not a lecture. Let the consumer ask as many questions as they need to. If you don't know an answer, say so—then find out and let the consumer and their carer know the answer.

Illness	Talk about the diagnosis and what it means. How was it determined? How common is it? How might the illness affect the consumer's future, and how might thinking be affected? Identify strengths to overcome limitations and how to think positively.
Health promotion	Nutrition, exercise, relaxation and stress reduction, minimisation of alcohol, smoking and other 'hazardous substances'.
Stress management	Talk about stress management and ways in which the consumer can manage their stress levels. Identify stress management techniques and strategies. Draw on the consumer's strengths and coping abilities. Discuss how high stress can lead to the worsening of symptoms.

Medication management	Adherence to medication is an important consideration for consumers to manage their illness. Discuss issues such as: how the medication works, what it does, what are its benefits, what are the adverse effects and how can they be managed, when and how often it should be taken, any foods/activities to avoid, and what could happen if the medication is not taken.
Stigma	Talk about the stigma attached to mental illness and how this is affected by the media. Identify strategies that can help combat and manage the stigma. Discuss how stigma can impact on self-esteem, and how the consumer feels the illness contributes to this. Changing self-stigma can help other people understand mental illness through acceptance and education.
Trigger factors	Identify trigger factors with the consumer and carers. If the factors which trigger certain symptoms can be identified, the consumer will be more able to prevent these from occurring and early intervention can occur.
Working together	Discuss how you, the clinician and the consumer will work together. Will the consumer have a 'case manager'? How will this person be chosen? Does the consumer have a say in who their 'case manager' will be?

Emergency department (ED) mental health triage

- ED triage aims to ensure that clients are treated in the order of their clinical urgency, which refers to the need for time-critical intervention. It is not synonymous with severity.[11]
- The ED triage nurse applies a triage category in response to the question: *'This patient should wait for medical assessment and treatment no longer than ...'*[12]
- ED nurses understand that clients will be seen in the timeframe that corresponds to the triage category allocated to the client.
- If you can't see the client in the timeframe, let the ED triage nurse know and advise when you will be able to see the client.
- ED triage nurses make their triage decision in 2–5 minutes, and sometimes less. Understand that they will not have all the information you may be expecting.
- ED triage nurses work in open, public spaces with little room for privacy. This sometimes limits the information they can get from clients.

■ TREATMENT ACUITY[13]
TRIAGE CODE: 1 = TO BE SEEN IMMEDIATELY
Description: Definite danger to life (self or others)
Australasian Triage Scale States: Severe behavioural disorder with immediate threat of dangerous violence.

Typical presentation
Observed: Violent behaviour, possession of weapon, self-destruction in ED, extreme agitation or restlessness—bizarre/disoriented behaviour.

Reported: Verbal commands to do harm to self or others, that the person is unable to resist (command hallucinations), recent violent behaviour.

TRIAGE CODE: 2 = EMERGENCY. TO BE SEEN WITHIN 10 MINUTES

Description: Probable risk of danger to self or others **and/or** client is physically restrained in ED **and/or** severe behavioural disturbance.

Australasian Triage Scale States: Violent or aggressive if:

- immediate threat to self or others
- requires or has required restraint
- severe agitation or aggression.

Typical presentation

Observed: Extreme agitation/restlessness, physically/verbally aggressive, confused/unable to cooperate, hallucinations/delusions/paranoia, requires restraint/containment, high risk of absconding and not waiting for treatment.

Reported: Attempt at self-harm/threat of self-harm, threat of harm to others, unable to wait safely.

TRIAGE CODE: 3 = URGENT. TO BE SEEN WITHIN 30 MINUTES

Description: Possible danger to self or others, moderate behaviour disturbance, severe distress.

Australasian Triage Scale States: Violent or aggressive if:

- very distressed, risk of self-harm
- acutely psychotic or thought-disordered
- situational crisis, deliberate self-harm
- agitated/withdrawn.

Typical presentation

Observed: Agitation/restlessness, intrusive behaviour, confused, ambivalence about treatment, not likely to wait for treatment.

Reported: Suicidal ideation, situational crisis.

Presence of psychotic symptoms: Hallucinations, delusions, paranoid ideas, thought disordered, bizarre/agitated behaviour. Presence of mood disturbance: Severe symptoms of depression, withdrawn/uncommunicative and/or anxiety, elevated or irritable mood.

TRIAGE CODE: 4 = SEMI-URGENT. TO BE SEEN WITHIN 60 MINUTES

Description: Possible danger to self or others, moderate behaviour disturbance, severe distress.

Australasian Triage Scale States: Moderate Distress if:
• semi-urgent mental health problem
• under observation and/or no immediate risk to self or others.

Typical presentation

Observed: No agitation/restlessness, irritable without aggression, cooperative, gives coherent history.

Reported: Pre-existing mental health disorder, symptoms of anxiety or depression without suicidal ideation, willing to wait.

TRIAGE CODE: 5 = NON-URGENT. TO BE SEEN WITHIN 120 MINUTES

Description: No danger to self or others, no acute distress, no behavioural disturbance.

Australasian Triage Scale States: Known consumer with chronic symptoms, social crisis, clinically well consumer.

Typical presentation

Observed: Cooperative, communicative and able to engage in developing management plan, able to discuss concerns, compliant with instructions.

Reported: Known consumer with chronic psychotic symptoms; pre-existing non-acute mental health disorder; known client with chronic unexplained somatic symptoms; request for medication; minor adverse effects of medication, financial, social, accommodation or relationship problems.

Medication safety

Medication safety is important for you and the consumer. Remember the six rights of medication administration:

- right consumer
- right drug
- right dose
- right time
- right route
- right documentation.

Also consider:

- right to refuse (involuntary status not applicable)
- right person administering
- right process followed
- effect of medication
- right outcome.

Medications need to be administered carefully and all precautions taken to avoid medication errors.[14] The following formulas must be adhered to.

Tablets:[15]

$$\frac{\text{Strength required}}{\text{Strength in stock}} \times \frac{\text{Volume}}{1}$$

Mixtures and injectables:[16]

$$\frac{\text{Strength required}}{\text{Strength in stock}} \times \frac{\text{Volume}}{1}$$

$$\frac{\text{Dose prescribed}}{\text{Dose in stock}} \times \frac{\text{Volume}}{1}$$

$$\frac{\text{Dose required}}{\text{Stock strength}} \times \frac{\text{Stock quantity}}{1}$$

■ WRITTEN MEDICATION ORDERS

- Generic name of the drug
- The dose ordered: *This should be in metric units and Arabic numbers (1,2,3)*
- Frequency
- Time
- Route
- Date
- Medical officer's signature

■ TELEPHONE MEDICATION ORDERS[17]

- Have the consumer's chart on hand.
- Document the following:
  - *date prescribed*
  - *generic name of medication*
  - *route of administration*
  - *dose to be administered*
  - *date and time medication is to be administered*
  - *name of medical officer giving the order.*
- Ask the medical officer to repeat the order.
- Read the order back to the medical officer.
- Get a second mental health nurse to hear the order and repeat it back to the medical officer as a second check.
- Make an immediate entry on the medication chart and note that it is a telephone order.
- Sign the order and have the second nurse countersign.
- Record in the consumer's notes.
- The medical officer should sign the medication chart within 24 hours.

■ MEDICATION DOSAGES

mL	millilitre
L	litre
g	gram
mg	milligram
mcg	microgram
unit(s)	international unit(s)

■ MEDICATION ROUTES

Gutt	eye drop
IM	intramuscular
IT	intrathecal
IV	intravenous
MA	metered aerosol
Neb	nebulised/nebuliser
NG	nasogastric
Occ	eye ointment
PO	per oral/by mouth
PR	per rectum
PV	per vagina
Subcut	subcutaneous
Sublingual	sublingual
Top	topical
VT	ventrogluteal

■ METRIC EQUIVALENTS

Volume
1 litre (L) = 1000 millilitres (mL) = 1000 cc (cubic centimetres)

Mass
1 kilogram (kg) = 1000 grams (g)
1 gram (g) = 1000 milligrams (mg)
1 milligram (mg) = 1000 micrograms (ug)

Examples of conversions
0.2 kilograms = 200 grams
0.2 grams = 200 milligrams
0.2 milligrams = 200 micrograms
0.2 litres = 200 millilitres

Drug scheduling system[18]

Drugs and poisons are grouped together in schedules. The Australian drug scheduling system below indicates drugs that require similar regulatory control over their availability.

SCHEDULE	DESCRIPTION
Schedule 2	*Pharmacy Medicine:* Pharmaceuticals that can only be supplied through a pharmacy. This category is for substances for which the safe use may require advice from a pharmacist, and should therefore only be available from a pharmacy.
Schedule 3	*Pharmacist Only Medicine:* Pharmaceuticals which must be supplied by a pharmacist in a pharmacy. This category is for substances for which the safe use requires professional advice, but which should be available to the public without a prescription.
Schedule 4	*Prescription Only Medicine:* Medicines that can only be obtained with a prescription. This category is for substances for which the use or supply should be by or on the order of persons permitted by state or territory legislation to prescribe (i.e. a doctor) and should only be available from a pharmacist on prescription.
Schedule 5	*Caution:* Substances and preparations which have a low toxicity level and require caution in handling, storage or use.

SCHEDULE	DESCRIPTION
Schedule 6	*Poison:* Substances and preparations with moderate to high toxicity. Accidental ingestion, inhalation, or contact with skin or eyes may cause death or severe injury.
Schedule 7	*Dangerous and Regulated Poisons:* Substances and preparations with high to extremely high toxicity, which can cause death or severe injury at low exposures. Schedule 7 require special precautions in their manufacture, handling or use. Special regulations restricting their availability, possession or use are necessary.
Schedule 8	*Controlled Drug:* Drugs of addiction. This category is for substances that should be available for use but require restriction of manufacture, supply, distribution, possession and use to reduce abuse, misuse, and physical or psychological dependence.
Schedule 9	*Prohibited Substance:* Drugs that have no therapeutic use, but are subject to abuse. Schedule 9 drugs are only available for research purposes.

Intoxication

■ STANDARD DRINKS

A standard drink is any drink containing 10 grams of alcohol. Drinks often contain more than 1 standard drink, but 1 standard drink always contains the same amount of alcohol regardless of alcohol type. A standard drink is a unit of measurement related to a particular amount of alcohol.

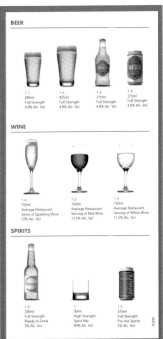

BEER

1.1
285ml
Full Strength
4.8% Alc. Vol

1.6
425ml
Full Strength
4.8% Alc. Vol

1.4
375ml
Full Strength
4.8% Alc. Vol

1.4
375ml
Full Strength
4.8% Alc. Vol

WINE

1.4
150ml
Average Restaurant
Serve of Sparkling Wine
12% Alc. Vol

1.6
150ml
Average Restaurant
Serving of Red Wine
13.5% Alc. Vol

1.4
150ml
Average Restaurant
Serving of White Wine
11.5% Alc. Vol

SPIRITS

1.2
330ml
Full Strength
Ready-to-Drink
5% Alc. Vol

1
30ml
High Strength
Spirit Nip
40% Alc. Vol

1.5
375ml
Full Strength
Pre-mix Spirits
5% Alc. Vol

■ FEATURES OF INTOXICATION[20]

SUBSTANCE	SIGN
Alcohol	Smells of alcohol, ataxia, slurred speech, disinhibition, depression, confusion, hypotension, stupor
Benzodiazepines	Slurred speech, sedation, loss of voluntary movements, nystagmus, low blood pressure, drooling, disinhibition
Cannabis	Conjunctival injection, anxiety, drowsiness, depersonalisation, impaired movements, confusion, persecutory ideation, hallucinations
Amphetamines/ Cocaine	Dilated pupils, increased P/BR/R and temp, increased motor activity, agitation, pressured speech, aggression, persecutory ideation, hallucinations, anxiety, convulsions, arrhythmia
Hallucinogens	Hallucinations, heightened perceptions, derealisation, depersonalisation, nausea, dizziness
Solvents	Ataxia, dysarthria, dizziness, sialorrhea (excessive saliva), nausea, vomiting, confusion, disorientation, hallucinations, respiratory depression, arrhythmia

Clinical handover tips

Clinical handover is the transfer of professional responsibility and accountability for some or all aspects of care for a consumer, or group of consumers, to another person or professional group on a temporary or permanent basis.[21]

Clinical handover should be clear and focused, and the information relevant.

Mnemonics are useful for handovers. SBAR, ISBAR, ISOBAR, iSoBAR and SHARED are all handover mnemonics. The choice of handover mnemonic should be fit for the purpose for the local context.

■ ISBAR[22]

I	**Introduction** *Identify yourself, role, location and who you are talking to* • What is your name? • What is your surname? • What is your position in the Health Service? • Which Health Service are you calling from?

S	**Situation**
	State the consumer's name, diagnosis, reason for admission or the current identified need
	• Why you are calling? What is the consumer's name?
	• How old is the consumer?
	• What gender is the consumer?
	• What are the identified needs/diagnosis of the consumer?
	• Is the consumer in the ED/ward or Community?
	• Is the consumer under the *Mental Health Act*?
B	**Background**
	What is the clinical background/history or context
	• What is/are the presenting symptom/s?
	• What are the current risks (self-harm, aggression, sexual safety, absconding, institutionalisation)?
	• What is the observation level?
	• What unmet needs does the consumer have to assist them at this time?
	• What medications is the consumer prescribed?
	• What allergies does the consumer have?
	• Any history of substance use/abuse?
	• How long has the consumer been in care?
	• Who is the primary carer and current level of involvement?
	• Current leave authorisations?
	• Current accommodation and discharge planning?
	• How did the consumer get to hospital?

A	**Assessment** *What are the current needs of the consumer (as identified collaboratively with staff and consumer)*
	• What is the consumer's current mental state? • What are the key MSE findings? • What are the immediate clinical needs? • What are the consumer's current risks and important observations/care levels? • What are the salient clinical signs that support the diagnosis? • What is the level of intensity of the symptoms, and how is this affecting the person's ability to function? • What was the result of the medical examination and key investigations attended/planned? • What are the consumer's vital signs (appearance, comfort, BP, T, P, R)? • What strengths/qualities has the consumer demonstrated? • What issues is this consumer currently working on, and what assistance have they asked for with goals (identified in care plan in order of importance)? • Summary of what the consumer has been able to accomplish. • What strategies have been used to increase this person's motivation to participate in their own recovery?

R	**Recommendations/request**
	What you are asking the person to do
	• Location for treatment, anticipated management and care.
	• Medications and what other teams should be involved.
	• Recommendations for immediate and ongoing care, with timeframes.
	• Changes in multidisciplinary team orders.

Clinical documentation

Effective documentation is a systematic and objective account of the care of an individual consumer and is vital for good mental health care.

■ THE SOAP APPROACH

The SOAP approach, developed by L.L. Weed in 1969, is useful.

S	**S**ubjective	What the consumer tells you the issue or problem is. That is, the consumer's view of their current problem or the issue in their words. The statement chosen should capture the theme of the interview.
O	**O**bjective	What the clinician observes the problem/issue to be. Objective information that matches the subjective statement. Descriptions may include body language, behaviour and affect.
A	**A**ssessment	Assessment of the situation, the interview and the consumer, regardless of how obvious it might be based on the subjective and/or objective statements.
P	**P**lan	Identify interventions specified in treatment plan. Should reflect need for follow-up.

■ EXAMPLE OF AN INPATIENT CLINICAL AUDIT TOOL[23]

Date:

Admission Date:

UR Number:

Diagnosis:

Contact/primary clinician on unit:

Treating Team:

Community Clinician (if case managed):

Audited by:

ASSESSMENT	Yes	No	N/A
Evidence of Intake assessment completed			
MSE documented			
AOD issues identified and assessed			
Alerts recorded			
Sensitivity label applied			
Diagnosis provided			
Information dissemination sticker completed			
Initial risk assessment completed			
Risk assessment updated weekly			
Medication Chart completed correctly			
HoNos completed			

Evidence of Consumer involved in treatment decision making process				
Evidence of Family/carer involved in treatment				
Provision of rights and responsibilities information				
TREATMENT & INTERVENTIONS				
Treatment Plan completed /Signed by consumer/ carer				
Evidence of Treatment Plan enacted				
MSE completed regularly				
Medical review/Consultant review				
Clinical review documented				
GP liaison				
Family meeting offered				
Therapeutic interventions documented				
DISCHARGE PLANNING				
Evidence of Discharge Planning				
Community clinician/case manager identified (for ongoing case management)				
Comments: (quality of documentation & evidence of planning)				

Issues Identified:

Quick relaxation techniques[24]

After working with a consumer on a ward or other clinical setting, you may notice they are anxious. This may relate to issues such as having a surgical procedure. Here are some techniques that might help them relax. Remember that different relaxation techniques appeal to different people. The clinician usually guides the session.

Whole body tension
Tense everything in your whole body. Stay with that tension. Hold it as long as you can without feeling pain.
Slowly release the tension and very gradually feel it leave your body. Repeat three times.

Imagine the air as a cloud
Open your imagination and focus on your breathing.
As your breathing becomes calm and regular, imagine that the air comes to you as a cloud.
It fills you and goes out.
You may imagine the cloud to be a particular colour.

Pick a spot
With your head level and body relaxed, pick a spot to focus on (eyes open at this point).
When ready, count five breaths backward: with each breath allow your eyes to close gradually.
Concentrate on each breath.
When you get to 1, your eyes will be closed.

Counting ten breaths back
With each count, allow yourself to feel heavier and more relaxed.
With each exhale, allow the tension to leave your body.

Transformations

When you think of images like…	*Imagine…*
Tightly twisted ropes	The twisted ropes untwisting
Feeling of cold, harsh wind	The cold wind becoming warm
Hard, cold wax	The wax softens and melts
Tense, red muscles	The red muscles soften or lighten to pink

Affirmations

Breathe deeply and slowly…
Let the tension flow away…
I am calm and relaxed, ready.
This discomfort will pass… let it go.
I have the power to handle this.
Relax the jaw, lower the shoulders.

Common abbreviations

ACMHN	Australian College of Mental Health Nurses
ACT	Assertive Community Treatment
ADHD	attention deficit hyperactivity disorder
AWOL	absent without leave
BAD	bipolar affective disorder
BPD	borderline personality disorder
CAG	Consumer Advisory Group
CAMHS	Child and Adolescent Mental Health Services
CBT	cognitive behaviour therapy
CMHT	Community Mental Health Team
CMI	chronic mental illness
DSM	*Diagnostic Statistical Manual*
DX	diagnosis
ECT	electroconvulsive therapy
EPSE	extra pyramidal side effects
FAS	fetal alcohol syndrome
FMHS	Forensic Mental Health Services
GAD	general anxiety disorder
HCV	hepatitis C virus
Hx	history
ICD	International Classification of Diseases
IDU	injecting drug user
MAOIs	monoamine oxidase inhibitors
MHA	mental health assessment
MHN	mental health nurse
MHPOD	Mental Health Professional Online Development
MI	mental illness
MS	mood stabiliser

MSE	mental state examination (sometimes known as mental status examination)
NGO	non-government organisation
NMHS	National Mental Health Strategy
NMS	neuroleptic malignant syndrome
NRI	noradrenaline reuptake inhibitor
OCD	obsessive compulsive disorder
PD	personality disorder
PICU	psychiatric intensive care unit
PTSD	post-traumatic stress disorder
RX	prescription
SSRIs	selective serotonin reuptake inhibitors
TCAs	tricyclic antidepressants
TCH	cannabis
Tx	treatment

Useful resources

Australian College of Mental Health Nurses—peak professional body for mental health nurses in Australia
www.acmhn.org

Beyond Blue
www.beyondblue.org.au; phone: 1300 22 4636

Black Dog Institute—specialist expertise in depression and bipolar disorder
www.blackdoginstitute.org.au

Headspace—Australia's National Youth Mental Health Foundation
www.headspace.org.au

Kids Help Line—confidential and anonymous, telephone and online counselling service specifically for young people aged between 5 and 25
Phone: 1800 551 800

Lifeline—24-hour telephone counselling service
Phone: 13 11 14

Mensline Australia
Phone: 1300 78 9978

Mental Health Council of Australia
www.mhca.org.au

Mindframe-Media—for media and resource information about suicide in Australia
www.mindframe-media.info

SANE—provides information and advice, 9 a.m. – 5 p.m, Monday – Friday
www.sane.org; phone: 1800 187 263

Suicide Callback Service—nationwide telephone support service for people at risk of suicide, their carers and those bereaved by suicide
Phone: 1300 659 467

VVCS—Veterans and Veterans Families Counselling Service—provides counselling and group programs to Australian veterans and peacekeepers and their families
www.dva.gov.au/health_and_wellbeing/health_programs/vvcs/Pages/index.aspx; phone: 1800 011 046

Endnote credits

1   Victorian Government, Department of Health (2011), *Recovery-oriented Practice Literature Review*, Mental Health, Drugs and Regions Division, Melbourne.

2   © Queensland Health (2005), *Sharing Responsibility for Recovery: Creating and Sustaining Recovery Oriented Systems of Care for Mental Health*, Queensland Health, Brisbane.

3   Mental Health Council of Australia (MHCA) (2012), *Fact Sheet: Statistics on Mental Health*, Deakin, ACT; (a) Australian Bureau of Statistics (2007), *National Survey of Mental Health and Wellbeing*; (b) World Bank (1996), *The Global Burden of Disease: A Comprehensive Assessment of Mortality and Disability, Injuries, and Risk Factors in 1990 and Projected to 2020*, Harvard School of Public Health, Geneva; (c) *Beyondblue National Initiative* (2006); (d) Orygen Youth Health, <www.oyh.org.au>; (e) Making Sense of Orygen Youth Health, <www.orygen. org.au/docs/INFO/MS%200YH2(1)>; (f) Mental Health Council of Australia (2006), *Time for Service;* (g) Australian National Council on Drugs (2007), *Drug Use in the Family*, ANCD Report.

4   Pawlik-Kienle, L. (2007), 'Signs of mental illness in psychology: Symptoms of psychological disorders', <www. suite101.com>. Reproduced with kind permission.

5   Neuroleptic Malignant Syndrome Information Service, <www.nmsis.org/index.asp>.

6   'Treatment' only: Nochimson, G. (2009), 'Toxicity, medication induced dystonic reactions', <http://emedicine. medscape.com/article/814632-overview>.

7   Cox, J.L., Holden, J.M. & Sagovsky, R. (1987), 'Detection of postnatal depression: Development of the 10-item

Edinburgh Postnatal Depression Scale', *British Journal of Psychiatry*, 150(6), pp. 782–6.

8   Black Dog Institute (2005), 'The Edinburgh Postnatal Depression Scale (EPDS)', retrieved from <www.shiregps. org.au/documents/MH_Edinburgh_PND%20Scale.pdf>.

9   Greenberg, S.A. (2007), 'How to try this: The Geriatric Depression Scale, short form', *American Journal of Nursing*, 107(10), pp. 60–69.

10   Patterson, W.M., Dohn. H.H., Bird, J. & Patterson, G.A. (1983), 'Evaluation of suicidal patients: The SAD PERSONS Scale', *Psychosomatics*. 24(4), pp. 343–5, 348–9. © Elsevier.

11   Australasian College for Emergency Medicine (2000), *Guidelines on the Implementation of the Australasian Triage Scale in Emergency Departments*, West Melbourne.

12   Australasian College for Emergency Medicine (2006), *Policy on the Australasian Triage Scale*, West Melbourne.

13   Australian Government Department of Health and Ageing (2009), *Emergency Triage Education Kit*, Canberra. Used by permission of the Australian Government.

14   Based on Glaister, K. (1997), *Medication Mathematics*, Macmillan Education Australia, pp. 56–57.

15, 16 Reid-Searl, K., Dwyer, T., Moxham, L. & Reid-Speirs, J. (2007), *Nursing Student's Maths and Medications Survival Guide*, Pearson Education, Sydney, p. 38.

17   Bullock, S. & Manias, E. (2011), *Fundamentals of Pharmacology*, 6th edition, Pearson Australia, Sydney, p. 28.

18   The Pharmacy Guild of Australia, <www.guild.org.au/iwov resources/documents/The_Guild/PDFs/News%20and%20 Events/Publications/Fact%20Sheets/scheduling_system. pdf>; and Virtual Medical Centre, *Australia's Unique Medication Scheduling and Definitions of Drug Scheduling*. Fact sheet available at <www.virtualmedicalcentre.com>.

19   Australian Government Department of Health and Ageing (2009), *New National Guidelines for Alcohol Consumption*, Canberra. Used by permission of the Australian Government.

20   New South Wales Department of Health (2009), *Mental Health for Emergency Departments: A Reference Guide*, Mental Health and Drug and Alcohol Office, North Sydney, p. 42.

21   Australian Commission on Safety and Quality in Health Care (2011), *Implementation Toolkit for Clinical Handover Improvement*, ACSQHC, Sydney.

22   Adapted from New South Wales Department of Health (2009), *Implementation Toolkit: Standard Key Principles for Clinical Handover*, North Sydney, <www.archi.net. au/documents/resources/qs/clinical/clinical-handover/ implementation-toolkit.pdf>.

23   Mental Health Professional Online Development (MHPOD), <www.mhpod.gov.au>. © CADRE Design 2012. Reproduced with permission.

24   © Black Dog Institute (January 2007), *Quick Relaxation Techniques*, <www.blackdoginstitute.org.au>.

ADDITIONAL REFERENCES

Australian College of Mental Health Nurses (ACMHN), *Philosophy and objectives of the ACMHN*, <www.acmhn.org>.

Weed, L.L. (1969), *Medical Terminology Records, Medical Education, and Patient Care: The Problem-Oriented Record as a Basic Tool*, Case Western Reserve University, Cleveland, OH.